OR Nurse Notes

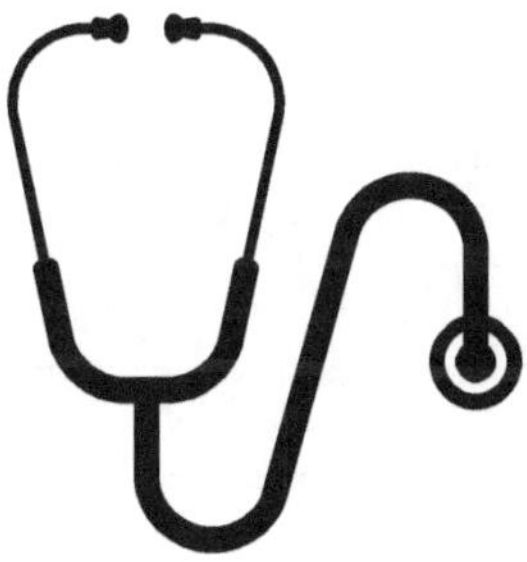

This book belongs to:

____

Coloring Section

I Had Fun Once, Then I Went To Nursing School

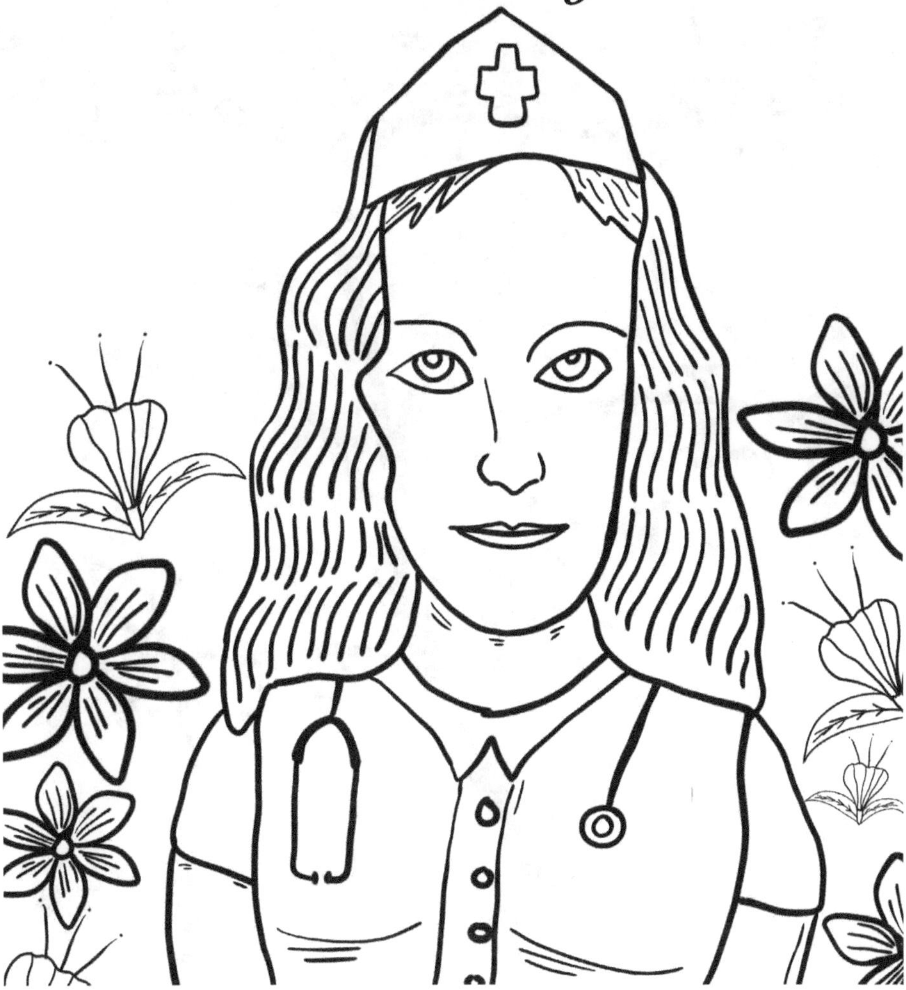

Ativan A Nurse's Best Friend

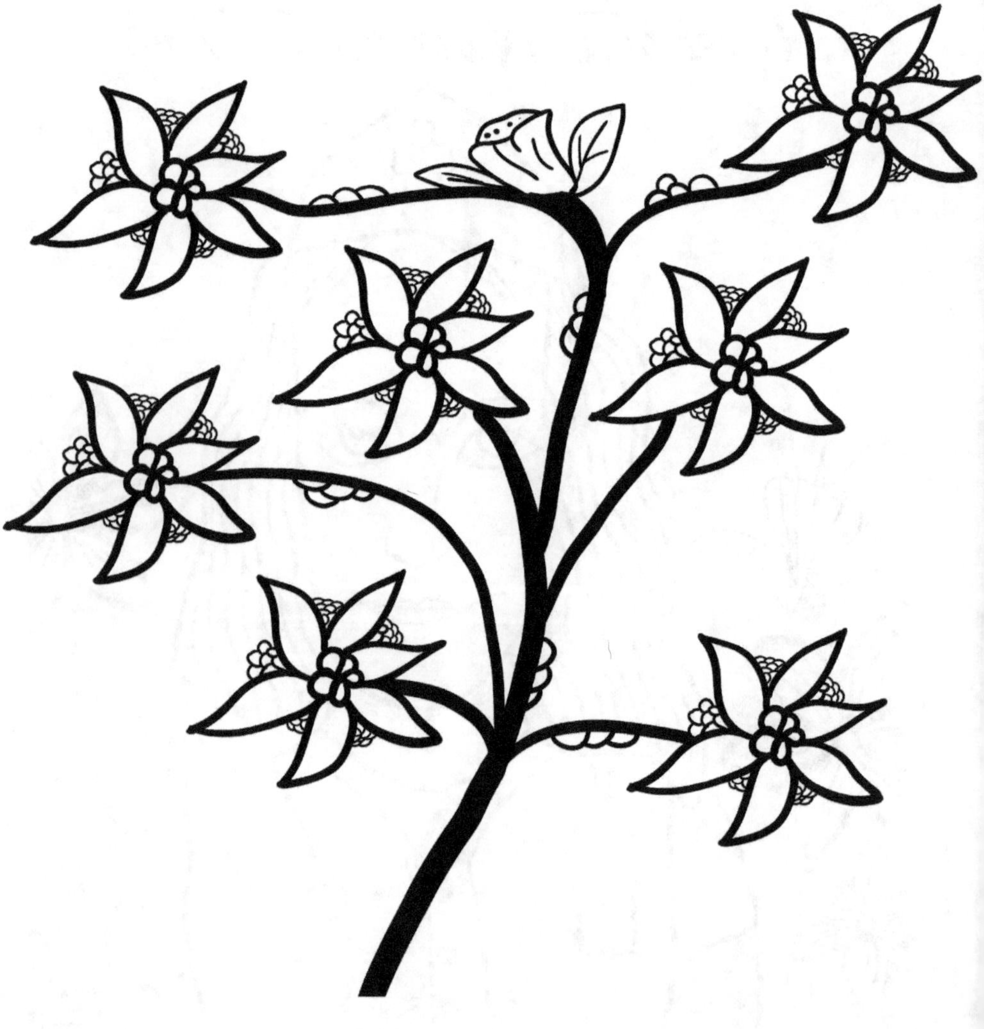

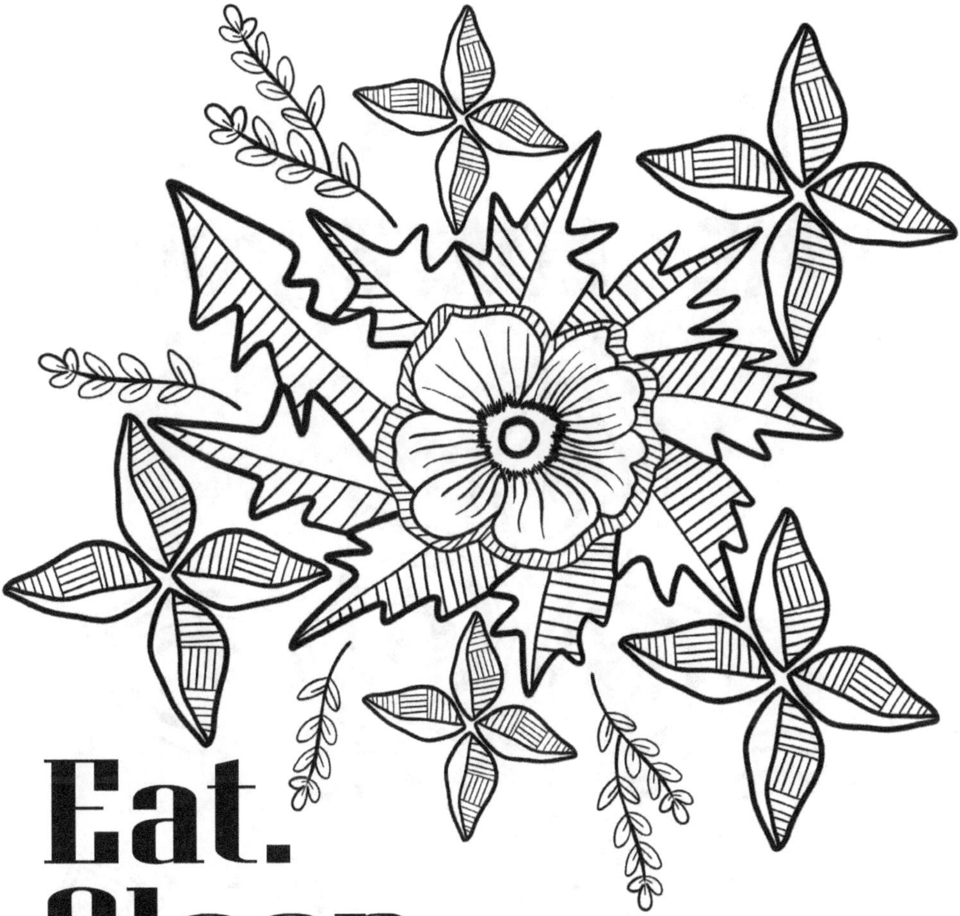

Eat.
Sleep.
Nurse.
Repeat

DO NOT MAKE ME SEDATE YOU.

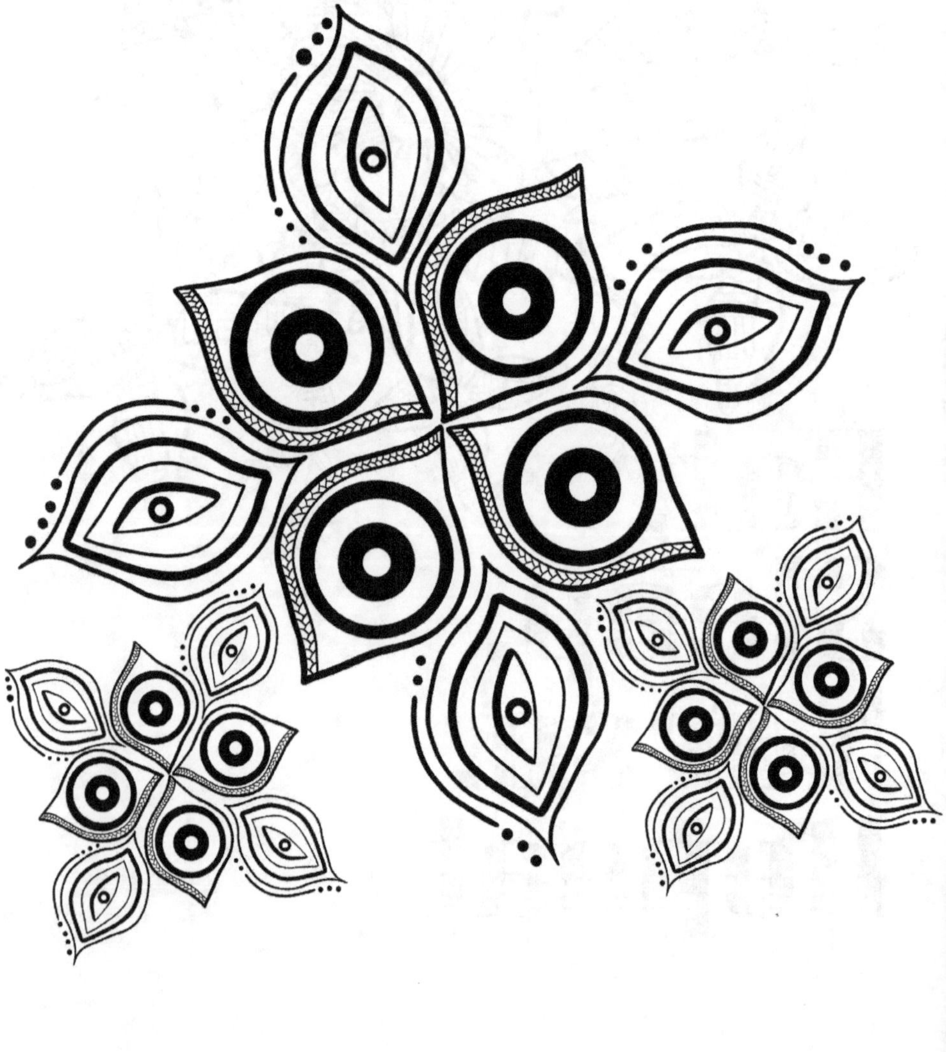

Best Nurse Ever

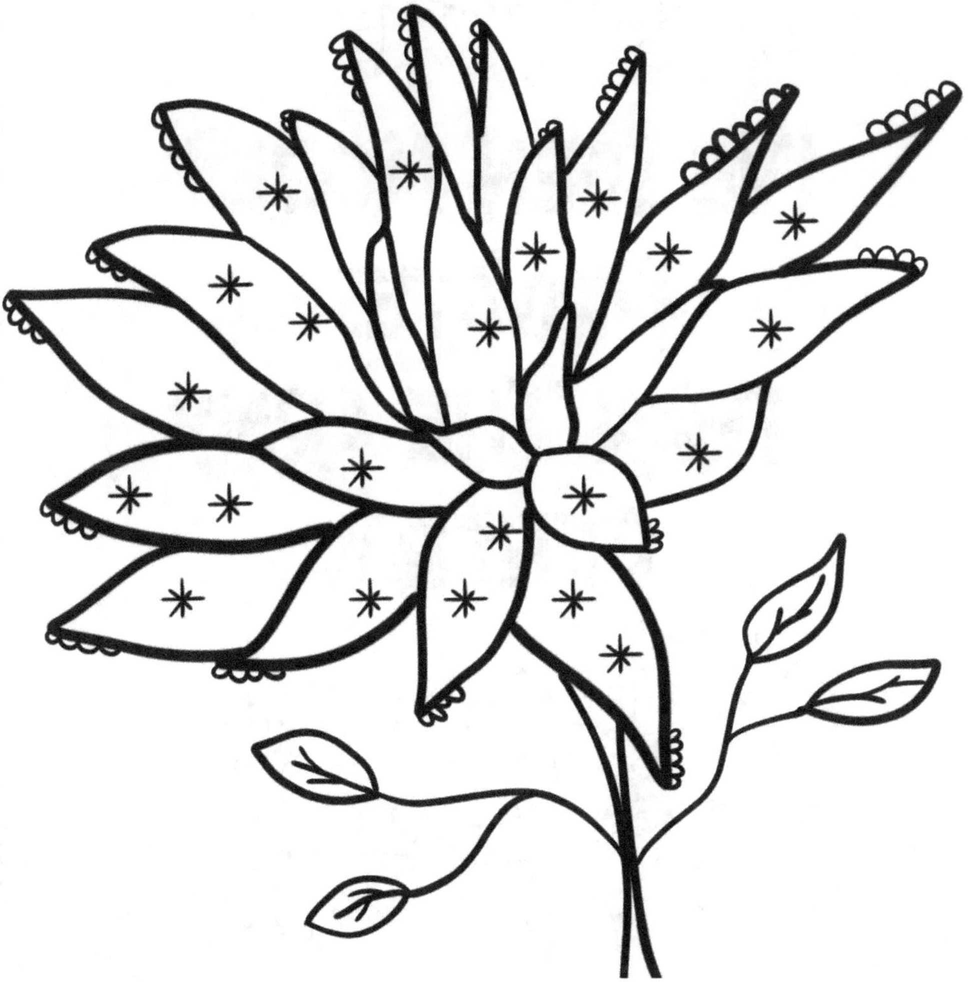

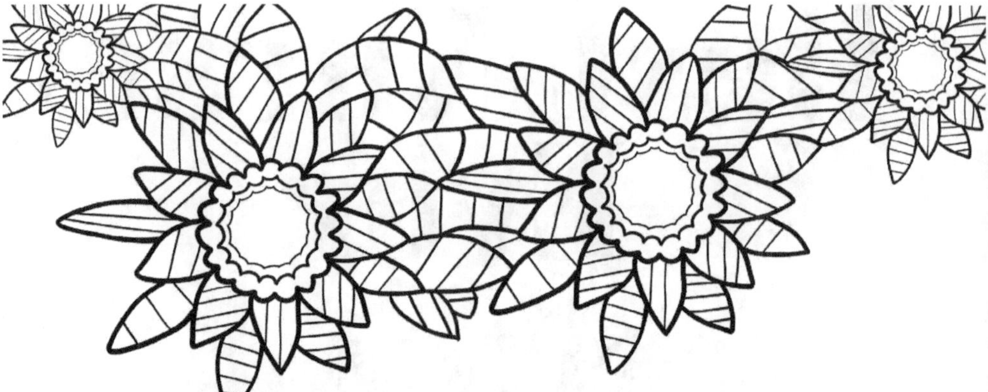

I'VE SEEN MORE
PRIVATES
THAN THE ARMY
GENERAL

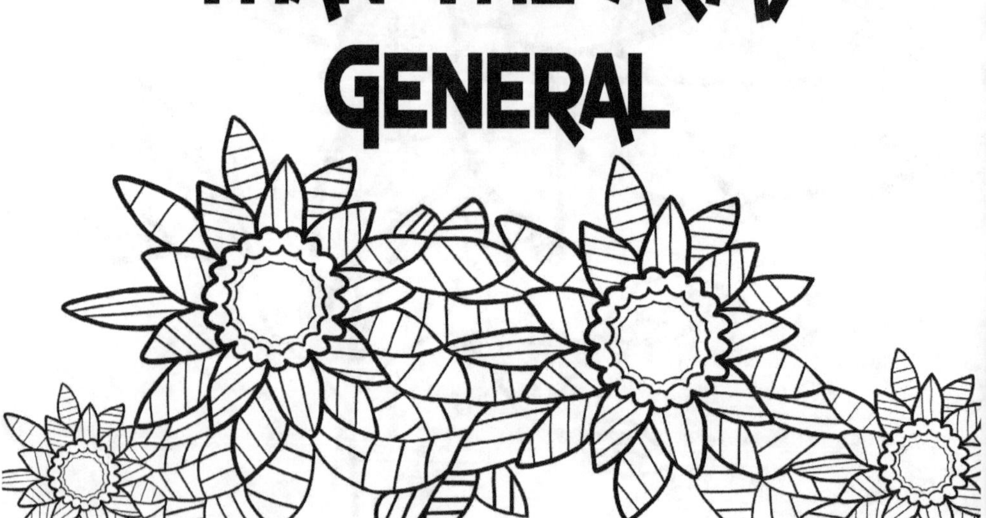

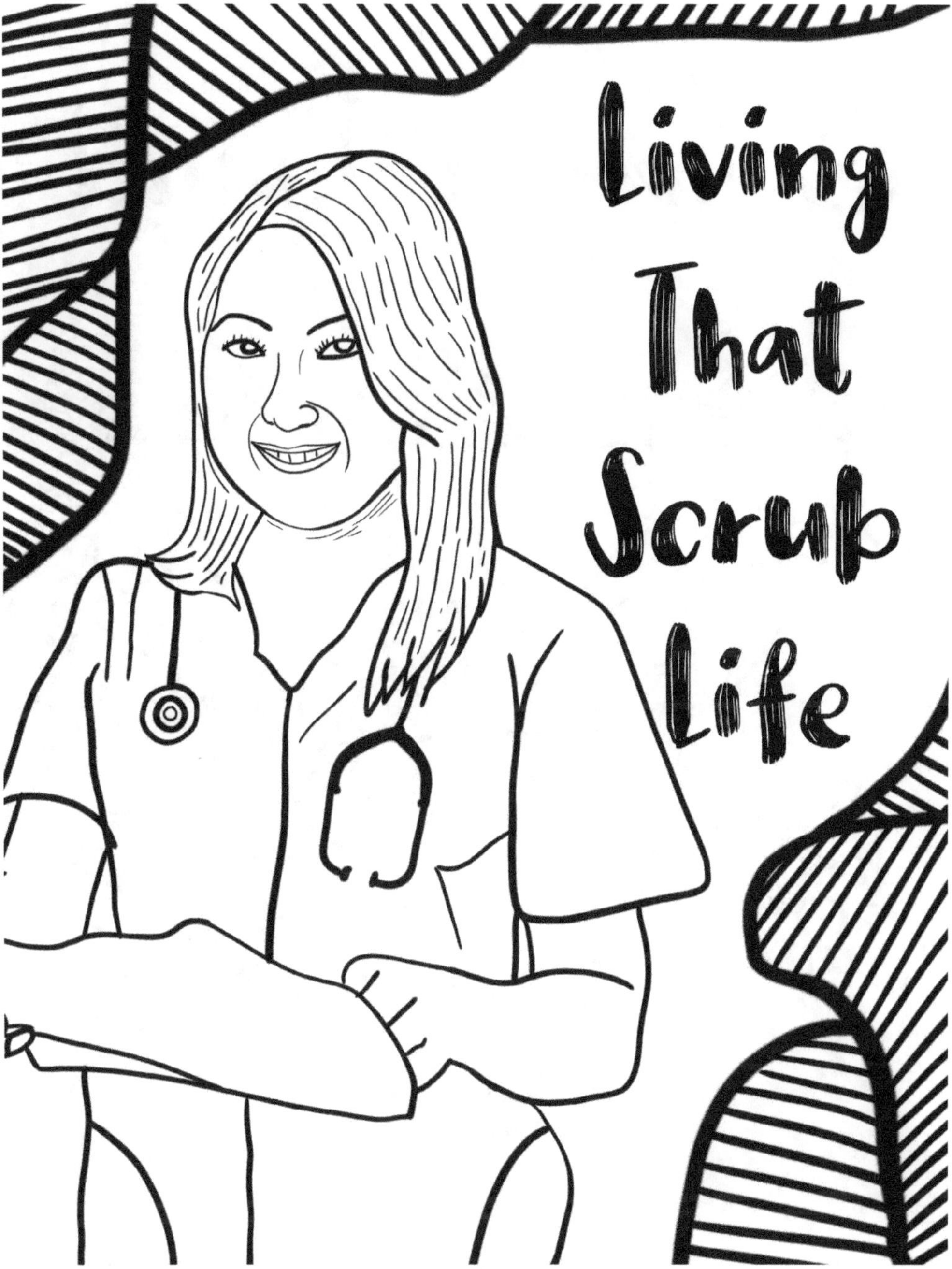
Living
That
Scrub
Life

Nurse Squad

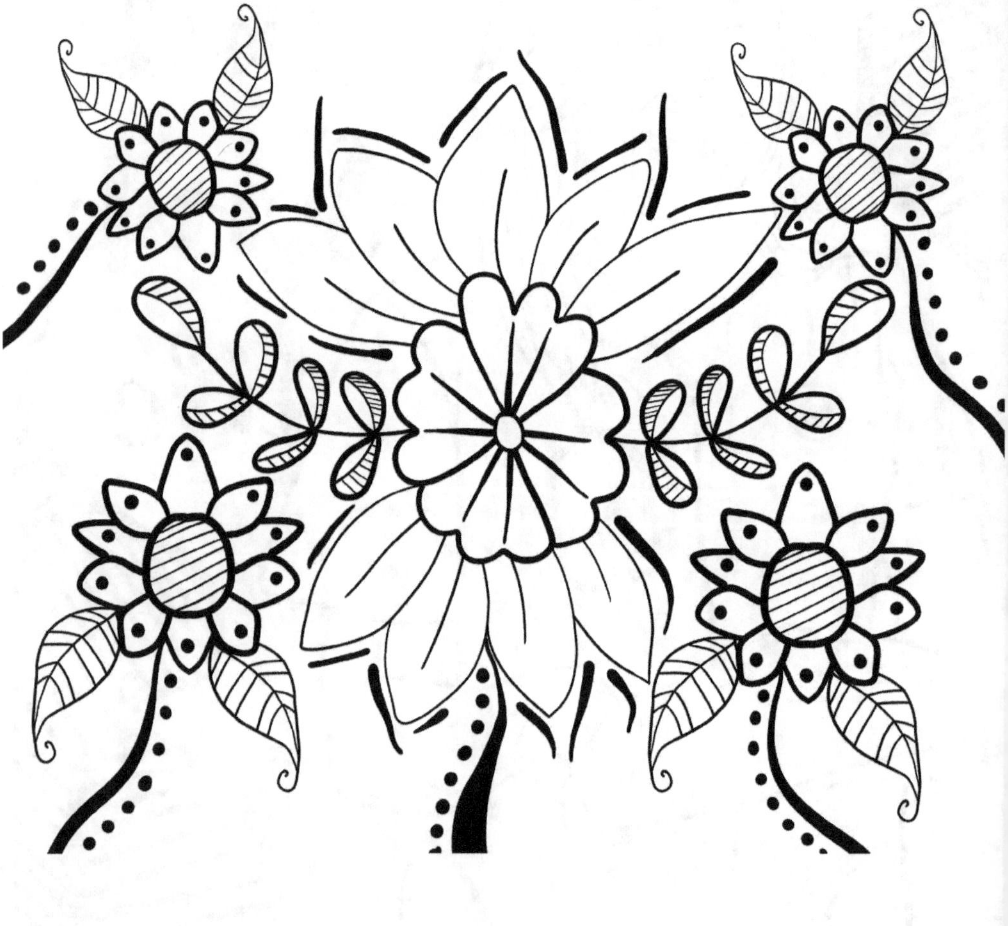

If You're Happy and You Know It, It's Your Meds

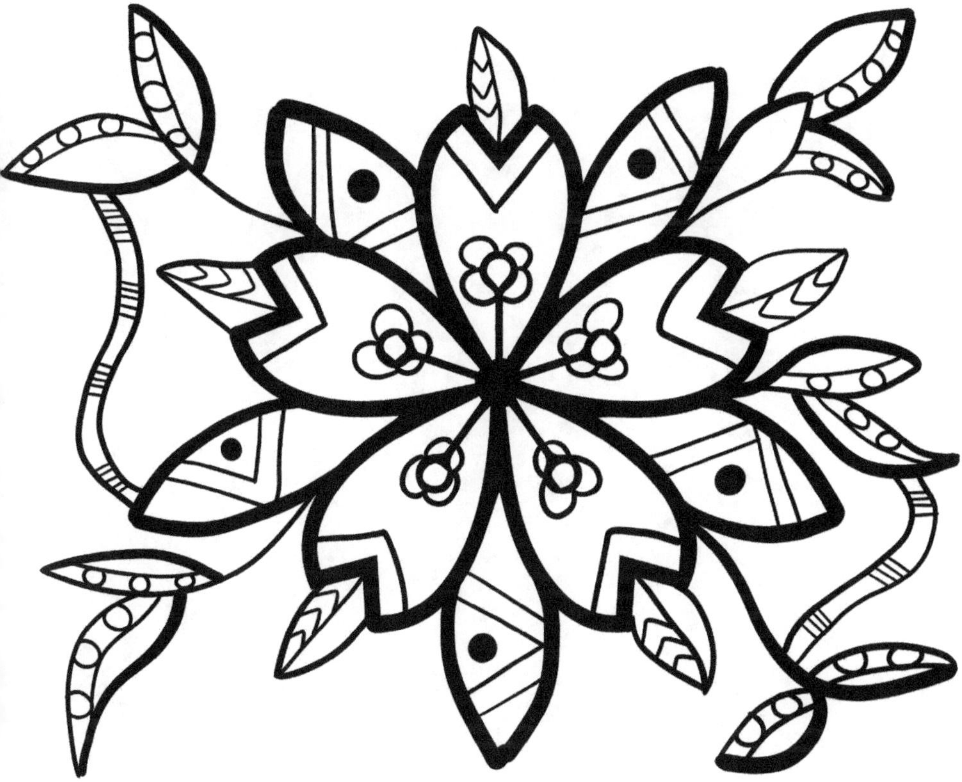

www.ingramcontent.com/pod-product-compliance
Lightning Source LLC
Chambersburg PA
CBHW072155170526
45158CB00004BA/1654
* 9 7 8 1 0 8 6 6 1 5 1 7 3 *